Ketogenic Fat Bomb Recipes

Table of Contents

Introduction 4

Savory **Fat Bomb Recipes** 5

Sweet **Fat Bomb Recipes** 10

Conclusion 37

Introduction

Into the Ketogenic diet? For those of you who do not know, when you hear ketogenic, it refers to a low carb diet in which the body produces ketones within the liver in order to produce energy. The basic end goal of a properly maintained keto diet is when your body can be forced in this metabolic state. When in the ketogenic diet, you will only consume roughly 75% of healthy fat and with a percentage of that amount it can be very challenging to keep up with.

You may receive low energy levels while on this diet, but rest assured that there is a solution for easy-to-make, energy balls for all keto lovers out there!

Say hello to the Ketogenic Fat Bombs, these snacks or desserts is high fat and not to mention delicious too! Whether you are craving to eat and too exhausted to cook something up or if you just may be looking to eat something sweet in a keto diet, this is the solution.

If you have not heard of a Ketogenic Fat Bomb, then it is about time you do! These fat bombs are a combination of ingredients usually from butter, coconut oil, some seeds and nuts and, of course, since they're called Ketogenic Fat Bombs, they are designed to follow the keto diet.

When you eat fat sources on its own, it isn't palatable and usually doesn't contain any protein or fiber. This is where the fat bomb recipes come in: all the high fat that you need in order to stay within your keto diet with higher levels of nutrition along with its delicious taste.

These fat bombs have to be made from scratch and with this eBook you are provided 25 different keto fat bomb recipes you can imagine, ranging from both sweet to savory!

Get your culinary gloves on.

Savory Fat Bomb Recipes

Bacon & Egg Fat Bombs

Ingredients:

- 2 large eggs (*preferably free-range or organic*)
- ¼ cup butter or ghee (*should be room temperature*)
- 2 tablespoons mayonnaise
- Freshly ground black pepper
- ¼ tsp salt (*to taste*)
- 4 large slices of bacon

Instructions:

Bacon

1. Pre-heat oven to 190C (375F), with a baking tray line it with baking paper and lay bacon strips out flat on the baking paper. Make sure not to overlap.
2. Once done, place the bacon-baking tray in the oven and allow cooking for about 10 – 15 minutes until it looks golden brown.
3. Once golden brown, remove from oven and set aside to allow it to cool down.
4. When cooled, crumble into smaller pieces for the 'breading' process.

Boiling Eggs

1. Fill a saucepan with water, maybe around up to three quarters and add a pinch of salt, in order to prevent from cracking.
2. Bring to boil and for hard-boiled eggs it should be cooked around 10 minutes.
3. Using a spoon, spoon the egg out of the water and place into a bowl of cold water.
4. When chilled, peel off the shells.
5. Cut up butter in a bowl. Add the peeled eggs into the bowl and mash it up.

6. Add mayonnaise, bacon grease from the baking tray previously and salt and pepper for seasoning and mix well.
7. Place in the fridge for 20 – 30 minutes so it can easily form fat bombs.

Fat Bombs

1. With the cooled egg mixture in a bowl and crumbled bacon in one use a spoon or if you have an ice-cream scooper.
2. Roll the eggs in a ball and place it into the crumbled bacon bowl and then onto a tray that should fit the fridge size and store it (*For up to 5 days only*).
3. OR you can eat it right away.

Ingredients:

- ½ large avocado (*about 100 g or 3.5 ounces*)
- ¼ cup butter or ghee, at room temperature
- 2 cloves of garlic, crushed
- 1 small chili pepper, finely chopped
- ½ small white onion (*about 35 g or 1.2 ounces*)
- 1 tablespoon fresh lime juice (¼ lime)
- Salt to taste (¼ *should do*)
- 1-2 tablespoon freshly chopped cilantro
- 4 large slicers of bacon (*about 120 g or 4.2 ounces*)

Instructions:

Bacon

1. Preheat the oven to 190C (375F), with a baking tray line it with baking paper. Lie over bacon strips and make sure not to overlap them.
2. Place the tray in the oven for around 10 – 15 minutes, until it turns golden brown.
3. Once cooked, place on the side and cool down.
4. When cooled, crumble the bacon into little pieces and place in a bowl for later.

Guacamole

1. Get the avocado, chili pepper, butter, lime, crushed garlic and lime juice ready.
2. With the avocados, you simply just slice, deseed and peel the avocados.
3. Cut the butter in slices.
4. Place all the ingredients into a bowl and using a masher or fork, combine it altogether well.
5. Once combined well, place the diced onions and continue to mix well.
6. Pour in the bacon grease from previously and mix again.

7. Cover with a foil and place in the fridge from 20 – 30 minutes.

Fat Bomb

1. Take the mashed guacamole and the bowl of bacon.
2. Start creating balls using a spoon or ice-cream scooper with your guacamole (*6 should do with every bowl of guacamole*).
3. Roll the balls over the crumbled bacon 'breading' and place in a tray that could fit your fridge.
4. Enjoy!

Ingredients:

- ½ cup of full-fat cream cheese (*100 g or 3.5 ounces*)
- ¼ cup of butter or ghee, at room temperature
- 2-3 tablespoon of freshly chopped basil, thyme and oregano (*or one teaspoon of dried herbs*)
- 4 pieces of sun-dried tomatoes (*drained and should weigh around 12g or 0.4 ounces*)
- 4 pieces of pitted olives (*any type at 12 g or 0.4 ounces*)
- 2 cloves of garlic, crushed
- Freshly grounded black pepper
- Salt to taste (¼ *amount should do*)
- 5 tablespoon grated parmesan cheese (*25 g or 0.9 ounces*)

Instructions:

Mediterranean Mix

1. Cut the butter into small pieces along with the cream cheese and leave in the table for about 20 – 30 minutes to allow to soften.
2. Mash it with a fork once soft and mix well.
3. Add the chopped sun-dried tomatoes and the chopped olives and mix well.
4. Add the freshly chopped (*or dried*) tomatoes, crushed garlic and season it with your garlic and peppers.
5. Mix well and place in fridge for around 20 – 30 minutes to harden.
6. Once hardened, take it outside of the fridge and start making balls using a spoon or an ice-cream scooper.
7. Place the parmesan in a bowl or on the table (*If you don't mind the mess*).
8. Roll the balls into the Parmesan cheese and place on a plate to either eat now or for later! (*It can only be contained to up to a week*).

Sweet Fat Bomb Recipes

Sugar-free No Bake Raspberry Cheesecake Truffles

Ingredients:

- 8 ounces of softened cream cheese
- ½ cup of powdered swerve (*erythritol or other sugar substitute could do*)
- 2 tablespoon of heavy cream
- 1 teaspoon of vanilla stevia
- 3 teaspoon of raspberry extract
- ¼ cup melted coconut oil
- 1 ½ cup of sugar free melted chocolate chips
- Pinch of salt
- Few drops of food coloring (*Optional*)

Instructions:

1. Using a stand mixer blend, place the cream cheese and swerve inside and blend until mixture is smooth.
2. Add the cream, stevia, salt, raspberry extract and natural food coloring until it has been mixed well.
3. Slowly add in the coconut oil by parts and blend on high until it is incorporated into the mixture.
4. Scrape it out of the blender and place it in a bowl for an hour refrigeration.
5. Using a spoon or scooper, scoop the batter into a parchment lined with a baking sheet (*You should be able to make at least 48 balls*).
6. Freeze the balls for one hour on a tray before coating it with melted chocolate.
7. When coating, just drop the balls into the melted butter one at a time then place on a lined pan.
8. Refrigerate for another hour and should be kept refrigerated until it is served.

Ingredients:

- 1 cup of unsweetened butter
- 1 cup of coconut oil
- ¼ cup of unsweetened vanilla almond milk
- Pinch of salt (*Optional if you have unsalted butter*)
- 2 teaspoon of vanilla liquid stevia or sweetener to taste (*Optional*)

Optional Topping: Chocolate Sauce

- ¼ cup of unsweetened cocoa powder
- 2 tablespoons of melted coconut oil
- 2 tablespoons of swerve or sweetener of choice

Instructions:

1. Slightly melt or soften the peanut butter and coconut oil together using a microwave or low heat on a stove.
2. Add the ingredients into your blender along with the rest of your ingredients
3. Blend it all until it is combined.
4. Pour the blend into a parchment lined loaf pan.
5. Refrigerate until it is set (*Should be about 2 hours*).
6. If you're using the chocolate sauce, just simply whisk all the ingredients together and drizzle over the fudge.
7. Make sure to keep it refrigerated and enjoy!

Chocolate Coconut Cups

Ingredients:

Coconut Candy

- ½ cup of coconut butter
- ½ cup of kelapo coconut oil
- ½ cup of unsweetened shredded coconut
- 3 tablespoons of powdered swerve sweetener

Coconut Topping

- 1 ½ ounces of Cocoa Butter
- 1 ounce of unsweetened chocolate
- ¼ cup of powdered swerve sweetener
- ¼ cup of cocoa powder
- ¼ teaspoon of vanilla extract (*Or you can use 3 ounces of melted sugar-free dark chocolate from Lily's*)

Instructions:

Coconut Candy

1. Line a mini-muffin pan and with 20 mini parchment papers.
2. Combine both the butter and coconut oil in a small pan over low heat. Stir it until it melts together and then add the shredded coconut and sweetener until combined.
3. Divide the mixture between the mini muffin cups and freeze it for 30 minutes until its firm.

Coconut Topping

1. Combine the cocoa butter and the unsweetened chocolate together in a bowl over a pan of simmering water (*Make sure not to have the bowl touching the bottom of the pan*). Stir until melted.
2. Once it has been melted, sift in the powdered sweetener and then the cocoa powder until its smooth.
3. Remove from heat and stir it with the vanilla extract.

Fat Bombs

1. Once the coconut candies have been set, spoon the chocolate topping over the candy and let it set for another 15 minutes.
2. Enjoy it now or store it in your fridge for up to a week.

Ingredients:

- 125 g (*or 4.4 ounces*) dark chocolate – 85% cocoa
- ¼ cup of extra virgin coconut oil (*55 g or 1.9 ounces*)
- 1 1/3 cup of chopped walnuts (*150 g or 5.3 ounces*)
- ½ -1 tablespoon of fresh orange peel or natural orange extract
- 1 teaspoon cinnamon
- 10 – 15 drops of stevia or healthy low-carb sweetener

Instructions:

1. Melt the chocolate in a water bath, adding coconut oil and cinnamon. Sweeten with stevia if you need to and mix it well.
2. Add fresh orange peel and to boost the flavor add some orange food extract.
3. Add the roughly chopped walnuts and mix well.
4. Spoon the mixture into a couple of small paper muffin cups or candy cups.
5. Place it in the fridge for a couple hours until it solidifies and store at room temperature.

Ingredients:

Crust

- 1 cup of almond, cashew or other nut flour
- ¾ cup of finely grated dried coconut
- 2 tablespoon of swerve or erythritol
- 3 tablespoon lemon juice
- 1 ½ teaspoon vanilla extract
- 4 ½ tablespoon of melted butter, ghee or coconut oil
- Pinch of salt

Filling

- ½ cup of softened at room temperature butter, ghee or coconut oil
- 1/3 cup of full fat coconut almond or other low-carb milk
- 1/3 fresh lemon juice
- ¼ cup of swerve or erythritol along with 1 tablespoon of sugar
- 1 teaspoon of sugar-free vanilla extract
- 2 teaspoons of lemon extract
- Grazed zest of 2 medium lemons
- ¼ teaspoon of salt

Instructions:

Crust

1. Grease 2 mini-muffin pans (*Should be 12 cup sizes*).
2. Combine the crust ingredients together and make sure to mix it well.
3. Place waxed paper on a straight surface and roll it into a log.
4. Cut it into 24 slices (*Should be 2 teaspoons of dough per tart*).
5. Roll each slice into a ball and press it into the tart pans.
6. Chill the crusts until ready to fill.

Filling

1. Place the butter or coconut oil into a bowl and beat it until it becomes fluffy (*You can choose to blend it with a food processor if ever*).
2. Add low-carb milk, lemon juice, sweetener, extracts, zest and salt into a bowl and beat it until the mixture is smooth.
3. Taste the combination and add more lemon juice or sweetener if needed.

Tarts

1. Spoon fill each crust with the filling and garnish with a sprinkle of lemon zest as an option.
2. Refrigerate until the tarts are set.
3. If ever you have extra filling, you can decide to make a pudding out of it or freeze it into mini-muffin pans to make individual lemon fat bombs.

Ingredients:

Coating

- 4 ounces of edible cocoa butter
- 2/3 cup of swerve or erythritol
- 1 teaspoon of lemon extract (*Other extracts such as Cherry would do*)
- ¼ teaspoon of Celtic sea salt

Filling

- 1 cup of swerve (*Or one teaspoon of erythritol*)
- ½ cup of lemon juice
- 4 large eggs
- 1 tablespoon of finely grated lemon peel
- 8 tablespoon of coconut oil

Instructions:

Cocoa Mix

1. Place the cocoa butter in a double boiler and heat it on medium high or until it becomes fully melted.
2. Stir in the natural sweetener.
3. Stir in the extracts along with the salt.
4. Place the combination into a truffle mold and allow to cool in the refrigerator until it has become solid (*About 1 hour*) or you can decide to make it quick and keep it in a freezer where it can be cooled within a couple minutes.

Lemon Filling

1. Combine the natural sweetener, lemon juice, 4 eggs and lemon peel in a saucepan and whisk it until it is blended.
2. Add the coconut oil.

3. Whisk constantly over medium heat until the mixture has thickened (*Try placing the mixture on the back of a spoon to test its thickness – should be about 12 minutes*).
4. Pour the mixture through a strainer into a bowl.
5. Place the bowl in a larger bowl that s fill with ice water until the lemon curd is cooled completely (*About 15 minutes*).

Truffle

1. Remove the mold from the fridge or freezer and fill it with the lemon curd filling.
2. Top off the filling with a layer of cocoa mix.
3. Place into a fridge to cool and set.

Cinnamon Bun Fat Bomb Bars

Ingredients:

- ½ cup of cut up creamed coconut chunks
- 1/8 teaspoon cinnamon

Icing #1

- 1 tablespoon of extra virgin coconut oil (*Not melted*)
- 1 tablespoon of almond butter (*Or double the coconut oil*)

Icing #2

- 1 tablespoon of extra virgin oil (*Or almond butter*)
- ½ teaspoon of cinnamon

Instructions:

1. Line a mini-load pan with appropriate liners (*You can use a different pan depending on your preference*).
2. Grab a bowl and with your hands mix the coconut cream along with the cinnamon.
3. Pat it into the pan (*Should fit 2 mini-loaf pans*).

Icing #1

1. In another bowl, whisk together the coconut oil along with the almond butter.
2. Spread this over the creamed coconut and place the bars in the freezer for about 5 minutes or more.

Icing #2

1. For the second icing, you just grab another bowl and whisk together all the ingredients for the icing #2 ingredients.
2. Drizzle the icing all over the bars and either freeze them again for future use or consume it.
3. With a knife, cut the bar into chunks.

Macadamia 'Fudge' Choco Fat Bombs

Ingredients:

- 58g or 2 ounces of Cocoa Butter
- 2 tablespoons of unsweetened cocoa powder
- 2 tablespoons of Swerve
- 112g or 4 ounces of chopped macadamia
- ¼ cup of heavy cream or coconut oil

Instructions:

1. Melt the cocoa butter in a small saucepan that is placed over a bath of water
2. Add cocoa powder into the saucepan.
3. Add the swerve and be sure to mix it well until all ingredients are well blended and melted.
4. Add the macadamia and stir it in well.
5. Add the cream and bring back to temperature, mix well.
6. Pour into molds or any paper candy cups.
7. Let it cool and then put it in the fridge for hardening.

Ingredients:

- 1 cup of extra virgin coconut oil (*200 g or 7 ounces*)
- 1 cup of raw cocoa powder (*100 g or 3.5 ounces*)
- 1 teaspoon of pure vanilla bean extract (*1-2 vanilla beans*)
- ¼ cup of powdered erythritol
- 10 – 15 drops of stevia (*Clear or coconut*)
- ¼ cup of chilled home-made coconut & pecan butter (*60 g or 2.1 ounces*)

Instructions:

1. Place the extra virgin coconut oil into a small bowl and melt it in a microwave on low heat for around one minute.
2. Add the raw powder, vanilla extract, erythritol and stevia.
3. Mix everything well and make sure there are no clumps left.
4. Spoon the mixture into any mold you desire.
5. Place the molds in the fridge for about 10 – 15 minutes until the chocolate is able to solidify.
6. Once it becomes solid, place ½ a teaspoon of chilled home-made coconut & pecan butter into the mold on top of the chocolate.
7. Top the remaining chocolate mixture on top of the coconut & pecan butter.
8. Place in fridge for at least 30 – 60 minutes until it firms.
9. Keep refrigerated unless being consumed.

Coco Walnut Bark

Ingredients:

- 2 tablespoons of liquefied coconut oil (*28g*)
- 1 tablespoon of unsweetened cocoa powder (*5.38g*)
- 1 tablespoon of powdered sugar equivalent (*12g*)
- 1 tablespoon of walnut halves that has been broken and toasted (*7.5g*)
- 1 tablespoon of heavy whipped cream (*15g*)
- Dash of salt

Instructions:

1. Mix together the liquefied coconut oil along with the cocoa powder, sugar equivalent, chopped walnuts and the salt.
2. Once mixed, whip in the cream and stir until the whole mixture is nice and creamy.
3. Spread it onto a wax paper (*About ¼ inch thick*) and refrigerate.
4. Once cool, snap of pieces and time to chow!

Ingredients:

- 1 cup of natural peanut butter
- 6 tablespoon of softened grass fed butter
- ¾ - 1 cup of powdered sweetener (*Such as Swerve and a little coconut sugar to make the sugar low*)
- 2 tablespoons of full fat coconut milk cream (*Refrigerate a can and just use the cream that sits on the top*)
- ½ teaspoon of vanilla
- ¼ teaspoon of sea salt (*Unless peanut butter is already salted*)

Instructions:

1. With a mixing bowl, place the butter inside and with a hand held mixer, use a stand up mixer to cream the butter.
2. Slowly add in the sugar at ½ cups at a time and continue to mix until it becomes fluffy.
3. Add the coconut milk cream and vanilla and continue to cream the bowl.
4. Add the peanut butter and salt (*Optional*) and continue to combine.
5. Spread the batter onto a baking dish (*Size would depend on the desired thickness*).
6. Refrigerate or freeze until the mixture hardens.
7. Store it into an air tight container in either the freezer of fridge.

Sugar-free Maple Fudge

Ingredients:

- 1 cup of organic butter
- 8 ounces of mascarpone or cream cheese
- ¼ cup of swerve
- 1 teaspoon of stevia glycerite
- 1 teaspoon of maple extract (*Or a few drops of maple oil would do*)
- ¼ teaspoon of ground ginger (*Optional*)
- 1 cup of pecans or walnuts (*Optional*)

Instructions:

1. Take a small saucepan and use it to melt the butter over a medium-high heat (*Until it turns brown and not black*).
2. Once heated, add the natural sweeteners.
3. Take out the mixture and place into a bowl for further mixture.
4. Using a hand mixture on low speed and once the mixture has cooled, add the mascarpone or cream cheese and blend until it combines.
5. Stir in the nuts and ginger (*If being used*).
6. Place a parchment paper of about 8x8 on a square baking pan.
7. Pour the mixture into the lined parchment paper.
8. Refrigerate overnight as it will allow the mixture to thicken.
9. Remove from pan and peel off the parchment paper.
10. Cut it into 1 inch cubes (*Should yield 24 servings*).

Ingredients:

- 1/3 cup of organic extra virgin coconut oil
- 1/3 cup of organic coconut milk
- ½ cup of swerve confectioner (*Or powdered erythritol based sweetener*)
- 1 cup of unsweetened organic finely shredded coconut
- 8 ounces of fark chocolate (*85% cacao*)

Instructions:

Bar Mixture

1. In a medium saucepan, combine both the coconut oil, coconut milk and the sweetener together.
2. Place over low heat and constantly mix until the oil has been melted.
3. Once melted, add the shredded coconut and mix well.
4. Pour the mixture onto a 9x5 inch silicone loaf pan
5. Press the mixture tightly and evenly to the bottom of the pan.
6. Refrigerate for at least 3 hours or until the mixture has solidified.
7. Turn the pan upside down and press the bottom of the pan so that the mixture will pop out.
8. Cut the mixture into the bar sizes of your desire.

Chocolate Sauce

1. Chop the chocolate into small pieces of equal size.
2. Melt 3 ounces (*85g*) of chopped chocolate in a water bath and make sure not to let the chocolate get too hot. (*Make sure to stir every now and then*).
3. Remove the melted chocolate from the heat and add the rest of the chocolate left over to the melted chocolate.
4. Mix every now and then so the mixture becomes smooth.

Final Bar

1. Dip the bars into the melted chocolate and place on parchment paper or cooling rack to allow the chocolate to set.
2. You can place it in a container to store for the next week.
3. Enjoy!

Ingredients:

- 75g or 2.6 ounces of softened coconut butter
- 75g or 2.6 ounces of softened coconut oil
- 25g or 0.8 ounces of unsweetened shredded coconut
- 1 teaspoon or 5ml of granulated stevia (*Or sweetener of choice*)
- 1/5 teaspoon or 5ml of dried ginger powder

Instructions:

1. Mix all the ingredients together in a jug until the stevia is able to dissolve.
2. Pour it into your desired silicone mold and refrigerate for 10 minutes.
3. Once cooled, take it out of the molds and into a container for either storage or consumption.
4. Enjoy!

Simple Lemon Fat Bombs

Ingredients:

- 200g or 7.1 ounces of softened coconut butter
- ¼ cup of extra virgin coconut oil (*55g or 2 ounces*)
- Lemon zest from 1-2 lemons (*Or use 1-2 tablespoons of lemon extract*)
- 15 – 20 drops of stevia extract (*Clear, coconut or lemon*)
- Pinch of salt (*Optional*)

Instructions:

1. While the coconut butter and coconut oil softens (*Room temperature*), zest the lemon.
2. Mix all the ingredients together and make sure all the ingredients are distributed evenly.
3. Fill up mini-muffin paper cups or with a silicone candy mold (*Which should hold 1 tablespoon of coconut mixture inside*).
4. Place it on a tray that can fit in the fridge.
5. Place in the fridge for 30 – 60 minutes until it solidifies.
6. Keep refrigerated or otherwise take a bite now.
7. Enjoy!

Ingredients:

White Chocolate Bar

- 2 ounces of cocoa butter
- 1/3 cup of swerve confectioners
- 1 teaspoon of toffee extract (*Or a few drops of toffee oil*)
- 1/8 teaspoon of Celtic sea salt

Milk Chocolate Bar

- Add ¼ ounce of unsweetened baking chocolate

Dark Chocolate Bar

- Add ½ to 1 ounce of unsweetened baking chocolate

Caramel Filling

- 1 cup of swerve confectioners
- 6 tablespoon of organic butter
- ½ cup of organic heavy whipping cream

Instructions:

Bar

1. Place the cocoa butter in a double boiler that is heated on medium high until it becomes fully melted (*Microwave is possible, place in safe bowl and heat on high for 1 minute or more until it is melted*).
2. Stir in the natural sweetener.
3. Once mixed, stir in the extracts and salt.
4. Place the mixture into a truffle mold.
5. Cool in the refrigerator until the white chocolate has become solid (*About 1 hour*).

Caramel Filling

1. Prepare everything needed for the filling (*You need to work fast or else the sweetener may burn*).
2. Heat the butter on high heat with a heavy bottomed 2 -3 quart saucepan.
3. Once specks of brown on the butter start to show, immediately add the swerve and cream onto the pan.
4. Whisk until the caramel sauce becomes smooth.

Truffle

1. Remove the mold from the refrigerator and add fill it with the filling.
2. Top off the filling with a layer of the cocoa butter mix so that the butter will be inside.

Ingredients:

- 1 cup of unsalted macadamia nuts
- ¼ cup of extra virgin coconut oil
- ¼ cup of grass fed butter (*Or use more coconut oil*)
- 1 vanilla bean (*Or 2 teaspoons of sugar-free vanilla extract*)
- 10 – 15 drops of Stevia extract (*Clear or Vanilla*)
- 1 tablespoon of powdered erythtritol or swerve

Instructions:

1. Place the macadamia nuts inside a blender and pulse until it turns into a smooth mixture.
2. Add the powdered erythritol and the stevia vanilla extract into the mixture.
3. Then, pour the mixture into the mini muffin forms (*Or you can use an ice cube tray*).
4. Place it in the fridge to allow to solidify.
5. Once refrigerated, you can keep it stored for up to a week or consume it. (*Don't leave it in room temperature as the coconut oil and butter softens*).

Ingredients:

- 1 ½ cups of coconut oil
- 1 1/5 cups of nut or seed butter (*Pumpkin seeds are recommended*)
- ½ cups of sweetener (*Any equivalent liquid or granulated sweetener*)
- ½ cup (*Or more*) of dried parsley flakes
- 2 vanilla
- 1 teaspoon peppermint extract
- ¼ salt
- Melted Chocolate

Instructions:

1. Melt the coconut oil in a small saucepan.
2. Add the left over ingredients into the blender.
3. With the melted coconut oil, place it into the blender until it becomes smooth.
4. Store it in the refrigerator for up to a week to prevent from softening.

Ingredients:

- ¾ cup of melted coconut butter
- ¼ cup of finely shredded coconut
- 3 tablespoons of melted coconut oil
- ½ teaspoon of pure peppermint extract
- 1 – 2 tablespoons of cocoa powder

Instructions:

1. Combine the melted coconut butter, shredded coconut, coconut oil and peppermint extract in a bowl.
2. Pour the coconut butter mixture into mini-muffin tins (*Only filling until halfway*).
3. Place into the refrigerator and allow it to harden within 15 minutes.
4. Remove the tin from the refrigerator and top each tin with the cocoa mixture.
5. Return it to the refrigerator until the chocolate is able to set on top of the coconut butter mixture.
6. When you want to eat it, just simply place the peppermint patty cups on the counter for about 5 minutes.

Ingredients:

- ½ cup of fresh or frozen strawberries
- ¾ cup of softened cream cheese
- ¼ cup of softened butter or coconut oil
- 2 tablespoons of powdered erythritol (*Or 10 – 15 drops of liquid stevia*)
- 1 vanilla bean (*Or ½ - 1 tablespoon of vanilla extract*)

Instructions:

1. Cut the softened butter in smaller pieces.
2. Place the cream cheese and cut butter into a mixing bowl and leave it at room temperature for about 30 – 60 minutes until it becomes softened.
3. Wash the strawberries and remove the leaves.
4. Place them into a bowl and start mashing them up with a fork or you can also choose to place them in a blender to smoothen the texture.
5. Add powered erythritol, vanilla extract and mix them well together.
6. Before you mix the strawberries with the other ingredients, make sure it is in room temperature.
7. Add to the bowl with softened butter and cream cheese.
8. Use a whisk or food processor in order to mix it well together.
9. Spoon the mixture into small silicone muffin molds or a candy mold of your choice.
10. Place in the freezer to let it set for about 2 hours.
11. Once done, unmold the fat bombs and place in a container for storage.

Cookies and Cream Truffles

Ingredients:

- 1/3 cup of chocolate protein powder
- 2 tablespoons of coconut flour
- 2 tablespoons of finely shredded coconut
- 4 tablespoons of canned coconut milk
- 1 tablespoon of dark cacao powder
- 1 tablespoon cacao nibs (*Or Paleo approved mini chocolate*)
- 2/3 cups of softened coconut butter (*For coating*)
- 1 teaspoon of softened coconut oil (*For coating*)

Instructions:

1. Combine all the ingredients into a bowl and mix with a fork except the ones needed for coating.
2. Spoon out the mixture into the truffle size of your choice.
3. Place the truffles into the refrigerator and mix together the ingredients needed for coating.
4. Remove the truffles from the refrigerator.
5. Cover the truffles with coating.
6. Return the truffles into the refrigerator for 20 – 30 minutes or until the coat has been hardened.
7. Store the leftovers in a covered container in the refrigerator.

Ingredients:

- 9/10 cup or 1 cup of blueberries
- 1 stick of butter
- ¾ cups of coconut oil
- 4 ounces of softened cream cheese
- ¼ cups of coconut cream
- Preferred sweetener

Instructions:

1. Place 3 – 4 blueberries into each mold slot.
2. In a saucepan, melt the butter and coconut oil over low heat.
3. Remove from the heat and cool for about 5 minutes.
4. Add all the ingredients and whip well with a whisk or stick blender (*Depending on which is available – the cream cheese will separate a bit, but it will still taste fine as a final treat*).
5. Add sweetener slowly and adjust to your taste preference.
6. Transfer the mixture to a pitcher for easy application into the molds.
7. Fill each slot with the mixture (*Be sure that it isn't fully to the top*).
8. Place in freezer for about 1 hour.
9. Pop them out of the molds and get ready for some grubbing!

Conclusion

Thank you for grabbing a copy of *Ketogenic Fat Bomb Recipes* book!

I hope this book has helped you in your journey of Ketogenic diet, especially in the area of preparing Ketogenic Fat Bomb recipes.

Finally, if you enjoyed this book and the recipes in it, then I'd like to ask you for a favor, could you be kind enough to leave a review for this book on Amazon? It'd be greatly appreciated.

You've got Ketogenic Fat Bomb recipes that will last you for days. So, let's get cooking!

Part II – Delicious Recipes for Fat Loss

One of the keys to success in the world of dieting is to not get bored with what you are eating. A good variety and good tasting foods are a needed for staying on a diet for as long as possible. Thankfully, we have recipes here that will get your fat burning and taste great. Let's start with the first meal of the day.

Breakfast Meal: Ketogenic White Pizza Frittata

Frittatas are great. A versatile breakfast meal, they are easy to prepare, easy to cook, easy to eat when you're in a rush in the morning and can be microwaved, reheated or even eaten just plain cold! All depends on your preferences. This dish is filled with fat from all the cheeses yet only 2g of carbs, this is going to make our body just burn all that fat from the cheese off.

For the recipe mentioned below, the cooking pan used is a cast iron skillet. But if you don't have one it can be just as easily prepared in a glass baking dish, however, if you do use that you may want to consider keeping it in the oven for just a bit longer.

Serving(s): 8

You will need:

- 12 Large Eggs
- 9 ounce Frozen Spinach
- 1 ounce Pepperoni
- 5 ounce Mozzarella Cheese
- 1 teaspoon Garlic – Minced
- ½ cup of Fresh Ricotta Cheese
- ½ cup of Parmesan Cheese
- 4 tablespoon Olive Oil
- ¼ teaspoon Nutmeg
- Salt depending on your taste

What to do:

1. Microwave the frozen spinach until it has been defrosted, this could take around 4 -5 minutes and then drain as much of the water as you can and set it aside.

2. The oven is then should be pre-heated at 375 Fahrenheit while you mix the eggs, olive oil, and spices into a bowl and whisked until all ingredients are mixed together.
3. Once mixed, place the ricotta cheese, Parmesan cheese and squeezed spinach (Break apart the spinach when placing into the mixing bowl) and mix.
4. Pour the mixture into your cast iron skillet and sprinkle all that good mozzarella cheese on the top and place some pepperonis along with it.
5. Bake it for 30 minutes or until the center has been cooked. (If you have the glass container inside the cast iron skillet then it would cook for about 40 – 45 minutes instead)
6. Take it out of the oven, slice it up and get ready to enjoy some good Ketogenic-style Frittata

Nutritional Value per Serving:
- 298 Calories
- 23.8 grams of Fats
- 2.1 grams of Carbs
- 19.4 grams of Protein

Benefits of this Recipe:

Spinach

It is no secret that leafy greens are good for you and it shouldn't be surprising that spinach (Which was the leafy greens that Popeye used to make himself big and strong) has numerous amounts of health benefits that will help your body fight against countless diseases, some of these benefits are:

- Protect yourself against inflammatory problems
- Oxidative stress-related problems
- Cardiovascular problems
- Bone problems
- Helps fight against cancer

Head to amazon.com to get your eBook copy of *Ketogenic Diet for Beginners: Start Your Keto Diet, Easy Recipes and Change Your Life!*

I'd like to share some of my other best seller books. They are best sellers in its category on Amazon. Simply head over to Amazon and get your eBook copy of the following:

- **Ketogenic Diet for Beginners: Start Your Keto Diet, Easy Recipes and Change Your Life**
- **Ketogenic Diet Recipes for Ultimate Weight Loss**